BIODYNAMICS OF OSTEOPATHY

Phase Eight

Second Edition

James Jealous D.O.

For more information about Dr. Jealous please visit:
https://BiodynamicsOfOsteopathy.com

BIODYNAMICS OF OSTEOPATHY Phase Eight

Hardback ISBN: 979-8-2955-3931-2

Second Edition 2025

James Jealous D.O. (1943–2021) practiced as an osteopathic physician, teacher and writer for many years. His life's work was to found and develop the specific methodology of Biodynamics of Osteopathy, following the lineage of Dr. A.T. Still and Dr. W.G. Sutherland.

This is one of a series of Biodynamics of Osteopathy books. They grew organically from sets of handouts written by Dr. Jealous and given to students during courses taught by him and his teachers. After many years he collected the handouts together and created individual course manuals, which he added to and rewrote many times. After several more years they evolved further into books.

TABLE OF CONTENTS

OSTEOPATHY IS SERVICE

We use our hands ...

To treat the Whole patient
To listen to the indwelling movements of Life
To treat all levels of illness
To assist in building the patient's functional reserve
To support homeostasis and trophicity by balancing the activity of the autonomic nervous system
To explore "laws not framed by human hands" (Dr. Still and Dr. Sutherland)
To cooperate and communicate with the Laws of Nature (Dr. Wales)
"To find the Health" (Dr. Still)
To get to the treatment plan
To get to the diagnosis
To help establish a point of Rest or Neutral around which the Whole can come to balance
To find Cause

We believe ...

We have an innate capacity to heal

The patient functions as a whole

The autonomic nervous system plays a major role in disease and healing

Structure and function are one form of activity

The Divine is indwelling

Life moves beyond death

There is a Constant Movement toward Normal

We are here to Serve Humanity

Normal is ...

"A sense of peace and harmony" (Dr. Sutherland)

Ease of motion, without tension

A capacity for Neutral

A sense of Wholeness to Life

The capacity for adaptation, change without compensation.

"Skill is proportionate to one's understanding of normal" (Dr. Still)

NOTE FROM THE AUTHOR

The trail ends here and begins fresh for the next generation. It has taken over twenty-five years to bring this to as much clarity as possible considering it is a living whole. I hope that the steps we have taken are useful. Osteopathy is an oral tradition, which can be threatened by rational agendas. It is a living irrational deeply instinctual science that gives us direction each moment we look for what we do not know in an endless Mystery of goodwill and service.

My bias is toward the incarnation of words that have arisen in the ancient past of man's history and are retained by sensation in the dictionary of natural and sacred phenomena. Will Sutherland was very specific with words and it was in exploring his language that this work began and continues.

There is something in Osteopathy that never ends. A lifetime is, as Tagore wrote, "a drop of dew on Lotus leaf." It seems true in its hugeness. Please enjoy all the love your fellow Osteopaths bring to the courses. That love is an Ocean of safety and peace for you to cherish.

James Jealous, 2019

Many thanks to Gregory Yesensky for his many hours of loving travail ...

THIS MANUAL IS DEDICATED TO THE FRIENDS OF OSTEOPATHY

To all the people who support the tradition without compromise. We stand together not to defend or promote, but to sustain something that cannot be partially pursued.

We did not understand, at first.

We came to it in ourselves as individuals, and not by dependence on words.

We came and we have forged steel from a whisper. We have died, rested, and started over. We cannot fail because we have no plan EXCEPT to Respond to the Tide.

There is Love here. It is not ours, we just happened upon it one day when we followed our Teacher's footprints to this Place.

In a spirit of Service.

"Twenty-four years ago, the 22nd day of June, at ten o'clock, I saw a small light in the horizon of truth. It was put in my hand, as I understood it, by the God of nature. That light bore on its face the inscription, 'This is My medical library, surgery, and obstetrics. This is my book with all directions, instructions, doses, sizes, and quantities to be used in all cases of sickness and birth, the beginning of man; in childhood, youth and declining days.'"
Still's recollection of his address on his sixty-ninth birthday

In *Autobiography of Andrew T. Still*

AN APPEAL TO THE THINKING OSTEOPATHS OF THE PROFESSION

Shall we permit the Osteopathic profession to be enslaved to the medical trust? ...

I unfurled the Osteopathic flag of freedom over forty years ago ... hold up the pure and unadulterated Osteopathic flag. Do not allow it to be trampled at the feet of our enemy. By winning this battle, we have delivered the greatest truth unfolded to suffering humanity. ...

Osteopathy is yet in its infancy. I have only brought forth the principles and truth that I have turned over to the profession, which has the wisdom and enough moral backbone not to offer any compromise with the enemy. ... If we cannot have the pure Osteopathic principles taught in our schools, I hope the faithful will rally around the flag and we will build an international school that will offer no compromise ...

Quote from a letter by Dr. Andrew Taylor Still addressed to the president of the American Osteopathic Association, Portland, Oregon, 1915, and printed in the 1948 American Academy of Osteopathy Yearbook.

BIODYNAMICS PROGRAM

To see the Health in another person, the overlay of tensions unrelated to the Divine Image must become Transparent. One does not look deeper, hoping to find something hidden. Transparency is the key to understanding. The art of seeing is not from personal effort, but rather from the action of the Tide upon your awareness. This expresses a Neutral mind, one not trying to see, but one silent upon the Stillness.

During his life, Dr. Still often referred to Mind, Motion, and Matter. Mind is the Divine Mystery, the Mind of Creation that animates Life and gives it motion. Matter is the Clay of Life that the Divine Breathes the Breath of Life into. The clay is the substance of the Dynamic Stillness, not the clay one sees on a riverbank. This Clay is Substantial.

Mind, motion, and matter once set toward incarnation are One. The Mystery that animates all Life unfolds its diversity in all living things. This Holy Animation is not man-made, not framed by human hands by science or art ... it is unlesionable, it cannot be destroyed, and it flows Eternally. It is beyond the veil of our self-centered senses.

Holy animation is called Love Eternal

When we sense this, our Zone A is transmuted, completely. We are suspended in Love.

In the first edition of *Osteopathy in the Cranial Field,* Dr. Sutherland collects his views and Dr. Still's into a picture that is clearly composed from beyond the veil of the ordinary senses.

"Motion must be guided and directed by a Supreme Being, down to the individual cell, or there would be chaos and death." … Sutherland continues … "Dr. Still understood the Cerebral Spinal Fluid as the highest known element in the human body; he envisioned this fluid as an intermediary in the movement of Divine Intelligence … A channeling of Creation into embryological segments and irrigating them with Life … giving form and function, order, and intelligence to our existence. Without this there would be only decay and chaos. All Life is manifest in this motion" (page 15, paragraphs 1 and 2).

Dr. Sutherland, on pages 15 and 16 of the first edition and in the April 12, 1948, writing in *Contributions of Thought,* brings out another Image of something beyond the veil of the anatomy. He describes feeling the Breath of Life (movement of Supreme Intelligence). He feels a Spark (fire) that is unerring, intelligent, and in command, superseding all other functions. He therefore called it Primary Respiration. Again we have an Image without anatomy or systems, which is moving perfectly (The Health). This was noticed only after he removed force from his observations.

He sees the interchange between Creator and Created (the patient).

All this is a picture beyond rates, anatomy, segments … just Creation, Fluid, Fire, Intelligence, Transmutation and Balanced Rhythmic Interchange … The Transparency to see through into this wholeness is an effect of being centered by the Tide. This perceptual maturity is evident in both Dr. Still and Dr. Sutherland.

RECOLLECTION

Doctor Still wrote:

"Solemnity takes possession of the mind, a smile of love runs over the face, the ebb and tide of the great ocean of reason, whose depths have never been fathomed, swell to your surging brain. You eat and drink; and as you stand in silent amazement, suns appear (where you never saw even a star), brilliant with the rays of God's wisdom, as displayed in man, and the laws of life, eternal in days, and as true as the Mind of God Himself."

Autobiography of Andrew T. Still (1987)

Being centered by the Tide began in Phase Four and has continued. We studied the effect of the Central Stillness upon our sense of self. We have entered the seams and found an Ocean that transformed us. We have found a living consciousness in the Ocean that expresses Love. We have found the perfection of the Health ... these events can merge into a single sense of wholeness that is universal ... it is very close to our hearts. It feels like one intimate family of all living things. Nothing is not alive! Invisible Beauty filled with Love for all, by all, in all.

PHASE SEVEN HIGHLIGHTS

Embryonic Breathing

Somatic sensation of the Tide passing through the House under the Sea

Awareness is transmuted by the Health

Liquid Light

Lesion as a precognitive act of the Health

Thoracic Respiration, Primary Respiration, and Ignition as One

Levels of Stillness and Silence reviewed

Neutrality of being

The Dying patient

THE THREE CIRCLES DIAGRAM AND COMMENTARY

The Three Circles schematically represent Osteopathic Thinking. These circles are real at one level and at another are overlapped in one universal wholeness. When we are oriented toward the lesion and its transformation, we are working from the bottom circle upward. This is the organizational pattern for the early phases ... from below upward. Once we pass into Phase Four, there is an effort to slowly treat under the Tide's guidance from the upper circle of wholeness, not following the lesion resolution at all. This, above all, requires waiting without any expectation and participating without goals like healing the problem. Trusting the Tide is the age-old challenge for our profession and ourselves as individuals. Embryology has, as a science, expressed a Mystery that operates the whole movement of life ... this should help our humility rise up ... but we are doers that must dream a little like we did in childhood ... study the Tide's precision and see its Beauty ... then Osteopathy will be obvious.

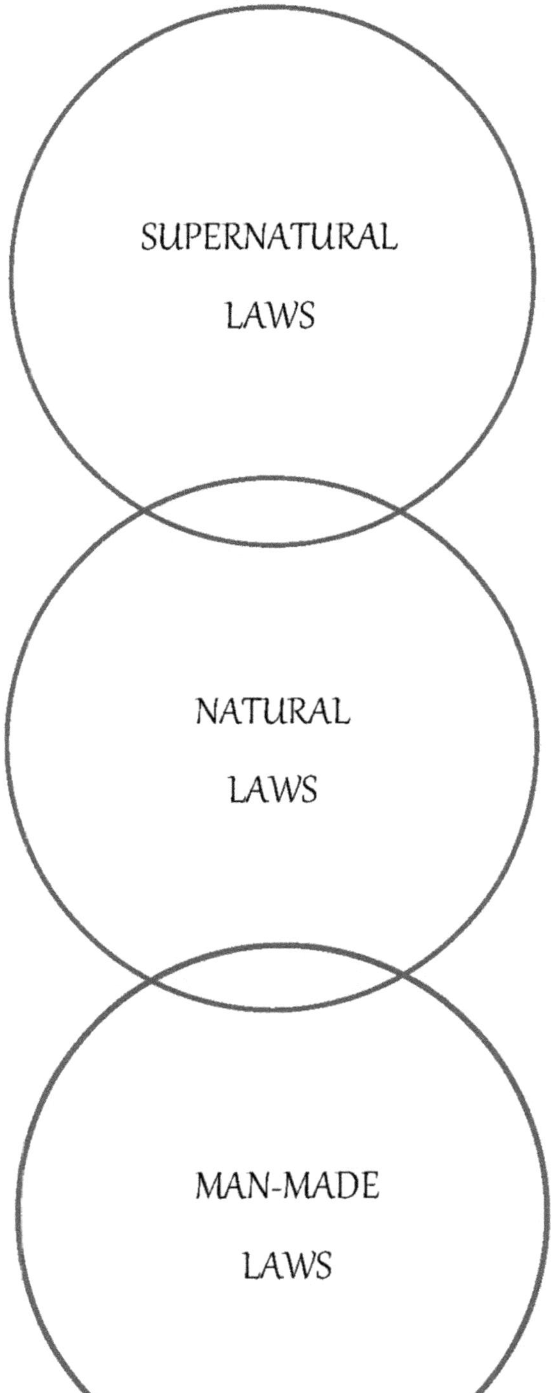
SUPERNATURAL
LAWS
NATURAL
LAWS
MAN-MADE
LAWS

WHOLENESS: A PRINCIPLE OF OSTEOPATHY

We have studied wholeness throughout the Phases. It is a living truth that challenges us. As Osteopaths, we claim to treat the whole patient. This comes true only after we separate the disease from the person and have reoriented our treatment to the person as an expression of wholeness. One huge step forward in this regard is to seek the Health in the patient as a doorway to the universality of the patient as an eternal expression of the Perfect. As wholeness appears in our awareness, it is obvious that the background has also moved into the foreground. What appears as material forms transparent to the wind of the Tide becomes the opposite. The living Tide dominates the awareness while forms move to the background.

This reversal of the senses is part of a spiritual awakening. One senses a wholeness in which the parts are suspended as expressions of the whole. But the visible world has been replaced by the invisible. All the diverse pieces are overshadowed by a moving wind of creation. One's response to this is usually fulfillment of the search for meaning, God, or inner child. The seeing of the visible/invisible as a continuum arises from Patience, which is the maturation of waiting.

Wholeness expresses the parts that we note as landscape and location. The parts have no input into the process of growth and development ... they are effects only. There is no anatomy in wholeness when seen in its wholeness. If we touch any point in the whole, it contains the whole ... a beautiful attribute of wholeness that lets the smallest be universal. This tactile reality is the reason we as mortals can touch the infinite in the patient rather than their lesion field. Few Osteopaths have integrated the whole into the sense of treating a patient's illness and yet the "cure" may lay in that historical residence.

The whole's boundaries are windswept and nonappreciable by human intelligence. The awareness of wholeness fills the observer with a love that ends all yearning for meaning or self-discovery. Our True Self is universal in its awareness, which means duality is dismissed as an illusion and love becomes the direction of ease for right action aligned with service and one's purpose in practice. The disease must not be identified with the patient as "who they are." One must search for the wholeness of life as the womb of conception and self-expression in which the patient meets a deeper reality than time and place. Osteopathy's magnitude must not be avoided because of the disease. The treatment of the terminally ill patient in Phase Seven proves this truth. Beyond anatomy is the power behind form and function where lesions cannot hide ... let's dig deeper and see what Osteopathy can really do.

WHOLENESS IN THE PHASES

In Phase One, we saw Neutral in the whole of Zone B. We saw it suffused by a Breathing that passed through the Neutral Substance as if it was Transparent. Wholeness is free of anatomy.

The wholeness we witnessed in Phase One was a unified singularity. One of the characteristics of Wholeness is a sense that there is one substance breathing. We felt transmutation cause the parts to merge into a single homogenized substance.

In Phase Two, we steadied our minds to begin the treatment with Neutral in the whole patient and then to engage wholeness through an Indwelling Stillness in the Fluid Body. As we did, Automatic Shifting occurred. We saw a connection between the wholeness of the Fluid Body and the Stillness that we communicate with. We came to the challenge of "sensing the Fluid Body as a Single Drop" ... this direction we took from Dr. Sutherland ... who said, "every drop knows the Tide" ... when we sense these words in action, we come to the wonderful sensation of the Wholeness. One feels and senses One Motion through everything ... and building as it Transpires. This Beauty is Wholeness.

Phase Three brought us face-to-face with the Wholeness of the natural world ... Zone D and the experience of the soft, slow movement of the Long-Tide with its Maternal Presence ... Mother Nature had to help us heal a little so we could feel an Ocean Breathing. We began to see a continuum between Zone B and the Sea Around Us ... sometimes Zone B would dissolve into the Sea ... a new sense of wholeness arose. As this new dimension of wholeness appeared ... we were treated ... as part of the wholeness ... the idea of just the patient being affected by the Tide during treatment becomes absurd ... whereas before we wanted only the patient to be targeted for exchange with the TIDE. Again our poverty of understanding was exposed ... Hopefully to our relief, Wholeness was getting more universal.

Phase Four was no retreat from the excitement of discovery. Phase Four was designed to help us be centered by the Tide ... as this occurred, the senses were transformed ... we began to see things differently. Wholeness creates all the parts and links them to a Central Midline. Individual Midlines are not a complete reality; each individual Midline is a single Fulcrum in a larger reality of Wholeness. Ancient civilizations appreciated these truths.

Phase Five was a pause ... time to integrate our changes in both perception and thinking. We entered Space, again another attribute of wholeness.

Phase Six was another pause ... more time to integrate. We dropped the attention and appreciated many new horizons. As the attention becomes an expression of the whole, unconditional love begins to express itself.

Phase Seven traversed the landscape of the images of the Health as we experience them during treatment and daily life. This sweetness and substance is so unconditional that it often breaks any false images of what Health might be.

WHOLENESS

Wholeness will grow on you ... it will transcend your mental agility... it will demonstrate Love as something Given equally to every drop of existence and not as something humans can "do." Maybe that's why we must "fall into love" and not be in love from our own need ... the difference is one of tasting the tension of the flow.

Around and through us is an Ocean. Empty the content and the wholeness will appear as a homogenized transparent sweet emptiness that is the essence of all manifestation.

As we have traversed the Pediatrics course, the whole has been revealed slowly: from Zone B to ... the River of Life ... and the Ocean as one place. Now we wish to divert our mind away from the known into the wholeness of everything. Our sense of this may come from many directions, but the key element is our neutrality of concept.

The whole is everywhere complete without distance or time delays. The center is everywhere. Its expressions are constantly dying ... pausing in the whole and returning to function ... we miss this because of our observer. The parts are floating in a nutrient and bio-kinetically appear as "place," but the real activity is in the Ocean as a whole, not in Zone B.

There is nothing to see in the Ocean, nothing. It is substantial basic space, transparent to Love creating each moment.

This means we can treat without knowing the specific lesion construction. I hope you have had the pleasure of watching the Tide treat in a fashion that contradicts your conclusions and demonstrates a clinical response that idles the intellect.

If not ... well ... work for wholeness with more conviction, discipline, and devotion, because the parts are expressions of the whole and nothing else.

Parts without the whole can never "be" at all ... nor can you fix them.

Please try that which your mind may believe is childish imaginings. Stay deeply imbedded with the science we know ... focus on resting your skill and insecurity. This perceptual death in yourself will synchronize your perception with reality and real science ... a Sea of sweet emptiness that is full of the "Master Mechanic's Hand" (A. T. Still) ... a Mystery that heals us all.

A CHILD'S SENSE OF WHOLENESS

Children's experience of wholeness is alive. For adults, the memory of this is limp.

Children feel a family circle and are intent on being in it ... often they bring the adults into this, and a new Zone B is felt by the adults that transcends the individual Zone B. We will discuss this as a topic and as a practice.

Children are very much aware of things that many adults search for.

When you treat, hold the child's sense of wholeness in your heart ... let it lead you to your own recollection and the spatial dynamics of the child's awareness.

Children also know the oneness of the spiritual family formed by all children ... they even have a universal language.

When we treat a particular child and are aware of all the children who will never be treated ... who have no access to help ... then we open a doorway to seeing into their world ... a little. There is plenty of love in the mechanism for everyone ... do not crowd the awareness of a child ... they can lead you without dismissing your help and treatment.

A LETTER ABOUT COMMUNICATION AND CHILDREN

Dear Dr. Jealous,

When my girlfriend found out she was pregnant, she had a dream that I was treating her and communicating with the baby.

She booked in and told me … I thought it was strange; I usually do not communicate with babies separate from the mom.

The first treatment at ten weeks was about moving through the fear, a lot of it—some mine, some hers, some from her social surroundings.

The second treatment, she was much calmer. It was a very deep and still treatment. The baby thanked me for looking after his mom.

Then he taught me what his hands feel like as an embryo. He showed me I still have these hands myself. "How can it not be if it once was?" he said.

Now when I am treating, I can really feel my hands as an embryo. I can feel the Wholeness and Oneness of this substance we are made of.

It is beautiful!

Beth

BREATHLESSNESS

One feels the Breath of Creation in oneself as the Center of Wholeness. The ownership of self dies, and one has the sense of being made, now. One feels the Unfoldment of oneself as one is Created.

Conscience ripens:

The Direction of Ease is a Compass of Divine Will; one follows.

The Body turns toward Ease and finds the Health.

The Soul keeps watching ... watching.

The Spirit and Body unite in conversations through sensation.

The Soul watches as its own will ... its power to influence ... is dying into another will.

What remains is The Passage to the Health.

When we see all this, we think ... "I am with my Health"... the sense of self shifts and we experience a certain healing from separation.

Love gets stronger, and the unresolved gets more central, deeper, more tragic. The wound opens as the Love Breathes ... we must use our Soul, our Awareness to detach from the fears and the pains. We must not touch these wounds or say "I" to them. We must step aside as if they are not ourself. We must let them see the Health without the shadow of our analysis or psychological interpretation or guidance.

We become Neutral to the effort to be anything. This Neutral allows us to see Wholeness in another way, as the vision, hearing, taste, smell, and being connect to the Health of Everything.

All "Healths" are One Health, breathed through by an Indivisible Love. There is no personal health, per se. The memory of this never diminishes. It is MEMORY ETERNAL.

The soma feels eternity as a sensation of complete Satiety and unites with Spirit. The soul watches and sees Choice and Free will. The Will to Respond ... or not ...

Wholeness is a word with no definition; only love is adequate.

Wholeness is Beauty radiant with Divine presence. Wholeness only exists in an Ocean of eternity that carries no sense of self into the I Am of God spoken in everything at once. The experience overshadows any attempt at definition. It is known by its presence and by its effect on the witness.

How does this fit into Osteopathy?

Osteopathy is grounded in the realization of a Supreme Intelligence creating all of life.

The embryology that I studied earlier in my lifetime has changed into a field of science that is proving to the rational mind the truth of Dr. Still's Principles of Osteopathy. Earlier in my life, I studied embryonic segmentation that gives rise to the integrative function of the Autonomic Nervous System as a whole. Un-lesioned autonomic function is indivisible—invisible but beautiful, often giving the observer a sense of tremendous peace and harmony, a peace and harmony that is not "in" the patient but through everything. Awareness of normal is a deeply spiritual moment when one's observer is burned away by Love. As we study the sensation of normal, we arrive at a point where palpation ends and sensing reaches deep into the Reality behind the processing of the parts. We come to an awareness of a homogenized whole, transparent to Cause. Our study of the dysfunction of the autonomic nervous system has allowed us to bring it to balance, and in so doing, exposed us to wholeness rarely sensed with any scientific tools other than our indwelling senses. Still said that our skill is proportionate to our understanding of normal. Over the years I have clearly seen the limits that I have placed on normal by my reductionist frameworks and fears of reaching beyond my limits. Since letting the Tide center me, I have found that all the fear has been replaced by love and dependency.

The great Osteopaths (those with exceptional clinical outcomes using only their hands) all point us toward this Beauty, this Wholeness. Generally, our professional groups are afraid and shun these realities. I have heard many voices that feel pain when these ideas are expressed. Many are angry at any idea that does not fit with their understanding ... this attitude is classified as neurotic and should be avoided by all of us. It has and is destroying the profession.

My personal despair with these voices was relieved by Bill Johnston, D.O., who contributed much to Osteopathy. He was a pioneer in communication with ease, wholeness, neutral, and indirect action. He did not like the direct approach of Dr. H. Magoun. Bill was inspired to find more healing with less mental and manual force. After I gave a lecture on the Death of Osteopathy, he was very upset with me ... he believed I was damning the profession. I called him and explained that the goal of the lecture was about accepting the death, not causing it. Our discussion was successful and we became very open and truthful with each other. I asked him to describe for me the end point of the perfect functional method of treatment. He was silent ... out of his silence rose a stillness ... a very deep and whole stillness, one that was familiar to me as a third level stillness. The pause between us was long. After a few minutes, he spoke. "You would not believe it," he said. I did not respond, as the Tide was still stilling me. Finally I said, "Thank you, Bill." The click of the phone faded in an air of love. He was a teacher, one that could take you into experience. In this case we went to a place of wholeness, the end point where healing enters the realms of what Still did and proposed to us. Bill showed me what we all have in common as Osteopaths. Where we all merge from our separate doorways and bias … He and I journeyed into a Common Ground beyond the entry point of our friction.

Wholeness is not a word with any meaning. The meaning comes from the witnessing of wholeness after a long and personal healing from living with the tides of life. Bill Johnston communicated wholeness directly. Functional methodology and Biodynamic methodology both seek to bring wholeness to the surface and transmute the veil that our lesions have created in ourselves and others.

Can we say that the hopeful end point of treatment is wholeness?

Yes … because the end point is beautiful and serene, and … No … because lesions are part of the wholeness, which is present whether we perceive it or not … therein is the reason why Wisdom cannot be captured by logic or definition, why there is a great Mystery in Life, and the more you know, the more you know the limits of being human.

PHASE EIGHT: MEDITATION

We have studied the zones for seven Phases; if normal, there are *no zones, only Wholeness.* Wholeness in our language means a sense of *all as one being-ness.*

All "Healths" are transparent to The Breath of Life touching soma with the eternal.

Awareness of wholeness ultimately brings us to the Divine Presence, Unconditional Love and Oneness or vice versa.

The message for today's meditation:

There are no Zones.
Begin with Zones A, B, and D…
Find each Zone, its center and its boundary.
Then find the place where they merge.
What happens?

THE HEALTH AND WHOLENESS

Eventually these ideas merge as our inner experience matures.

The sense of lesions and chaos in the world around us melts into a knowing that deeply expresses the truth we all seek. Wholeness incorporates all of life, not just human preferences. The unresolved Zone A, and the questions about how and why, all blend into a single reality where everything is sheltered by the whole and its presence. It is here we understand life in a loving manner.

At conception the perfect in its completeness enters time ... incarnates. Growth is toward what is already complete.

"It's the not-yet in the now, the taste of the fruit that does not-yet exist, hanging the blossom on the bough."

Laurens van der Post

The being-ness we seek is already here. It leads us forward by its scent, which is a yearning for being touched by the perfect. It is a loneliness unsatiated by things of this world. It is a silent voice. It is an inner child. It is the soul adoring. One cannot find the Health unless the mind is first transmuted by the Health; after we are healed, we see the Healer. This fact is easily overlooked because when we succeed, we do not always see that Transmutation comes into us, then we awaken. It can be so quick that we think we centered ourselves.

Now find the interface between your Zone A and the Sweet Warm Honey-like Substance of the Health. This is the Health treating you ...

where is the interface?

What percentage of you is connected to the Health? What percentage is not?

These percentages can be a guide of sorts; check every few months and see ... you will notice gains even when you do not believe you are changing.

THE BREATHING OF THE SEA AROUND US

The "House Under the Sea" became Dr. Sutherland's metaphor for the universal wholeness of Life.

The zones as we know them are tools to help us meet the Health in its natural setting, which is a deeply spiritual place with no parts. This universal space includes all of life. Its substance appears as nothing until we see the incarnate presence of its intention in the natural world. This universal wholeness is referred to by many spiritual teachers as the Great Ocean. It has a presence of Divine love and grace. In children we see this as their neutral landscape. Adults can touch it at moments. This zone is the "Sea Around Us" that is an Ocean extending infinitely and filled with Mystery.

This meaning comes directly from Still/Sutherland and refers to a real place.

Zone A begins at the central stillness and ends at the skin ... it is in the ocean but does not respond to it even though it gets fed by its Life force.

Zone B begins at the central stillness and ends in the Ocean (ideal). It can breathe with the Ocean.

Zone D begins at the central stillness and ends at the horizon. It is in the Ocean as the natural world. It is governed by instinct.

Zone C is one's sense of the spirit of the Ocean.

The Ocean has no parts and yet creates them. It is universal. The True Self abides here and is connected to its child in the natural world. This is called by us the inner child, which is our God-given gift of being designed to serve.

The unfolding of our form and function is a Mystery. We can, however, see certain relationships. One that is remarkable is the relationship of the Presence of Primary Respiration in the Sea Around Us to the individual fulcrums of specific functions. The Presence in the Sea is different than the Long-Tide or the Dynamic Stillness. In Phases Three, Four, and Five we studied the Long-ide and the Dynamic Stillness as therapeutic forces. Now we come to a new set of principles that reveal an essential relationship in healing. This relationship is about the Presence of the Sea, a living wisdom and love that creates our form and function. At first, it appears to be outside and the fulcrum inside of us, but the spatial sense of this will change as we work with it. Our True Zone B is the Ocean.

In the Sea Around Us there are no separations, only Oneness. The neutral here is everywhere. All breathing moves from a single cause in the whole. We will explore the meaning of this at different levels of separation and wholeness.

We begin by sensing the touch of the Ocean without moving our attention at all.

We will then check thoracic respiration, its fulcrum and its direction of ease.

Then we will do the same with primary respiration.

Then we will find the stillness they share and wait ...

Oneness is a child's world ... the Single Breath is called the embryonic breath.

Our consciousness is a gift; we do not own it.
If we control it, we lose Wholeness.
We become isolated from the Love and Sweetness of Creation.
As we let the Tide center us, we return to intimacy with an Ocean of grace.

Our Breathing shifts ... pauses ... and an Embryonic Breath appears.

THE FIRST BREATH

This commentary is about Osteopathic vital signs related to the First Breath and how that Breath creates momentum for present and future health issues.

Little is written on this subject, but the oral teaching has been passed on for decades. All the basic courses I attended (twelve) mentioned the First Breath.

The person who made the most sense to me was Dr. Fulford. He focused on the long-term sequelae in children who had not completed the First Breath, those who were desynchronized from the unity of all Breaths being One when we enter this world. From his direction and insight I pursued this topic in many ways ... I have studied it and used it in practice for thirty-five years ... it is very practical knowledge in spite of the spiritual overtones.

The first earthly breath of a newborn is always a moment of marvelous beauty and relief.

"The movement of the Breaths through the birthing as a Whole creates an individual, aligned consciously with the Health and able to function freely." These words coming from Dr. Fulford were few and valued.

What did he mean?

My understanding while talking to him was based upon my knowledge of the mystical path he had followed and what the words "whole," "individual," "consciously aligned," and "free-willed" would mean in the inner world ...

Children are remarkably complete, whole, and free. They unfold from the blueprint of Life set at conception. In order for development to unfold continuously, one must have a well-established fulcrum between Primary Respiration, Thoracic Respiration, and Ignition.

At the time of the First Breath after birth, the demands of life increase severely ... the Ignition creates more fire, the Tide is orchestrated, the Dynamic Stillness pours in through the Midline, and as the air rushes into the lungs, One Breath is set in time as Eternity comes ashore. The feeling is Wholeness, not parts. If one feels parts, then there is a lesion.

To be an Individual, in Dr. Fulford's terminology, means to follow the destiny of unfoldment, not worldly images. The journey for Dr. Fulford was to listen to the Love behind Creation and follow its voice. The result of this hard work would be that one becomes what God made them for, not what their genetics and ego might overlay.

The First Breath establishes Memory and the vital Oneness that carries one's Name. If the First Breath is weak, our struggle to know ourselves may be extended and spiritual maturity delayed (prolonging the sense of isolation from Life).

To be consciously aligned means, in the context of his work, to be aware of Divine Will and to have an instinctual need to be in the presence of Love and perfection. This is the Self of the Immune System.

Free will, as Dr. Fulford put it, is when one has no slavery to habits or beliefs. One is free to be shifted by the movement of the Creator's Hand. One is free to lighten the load of World Suffering. One is detached, impartial to everything, neutral and responsive to the unfoldment of God's Love. This is not a willy-nilly going with the flow ... it is love meeting Love with no preconceived outcomes. It is fearlessness in the face of one's timidity.

In the Biodynamic view, the first Breath is Relative, not Absolute. The First True Breath is at or before conception. Obviously thoracic respiration (O_2 metabolic exchange) begins much earlier than birth. The Birthing Breath is the first earthly breath, and ideally Thoracic, Primary, and the ignition move together as One.

Think about the capacity of Zone B to do its work, to accomplish unfoldment of the blueprint of Life, if the First Breath is desynchronized and weakened. It cannot follow the outpouring of the movement of Life as it grows, if it has no power to do so. The first hint of inertia, if you are not trained to see it through the fluid body dynamics, is slowness in the remolding of the head after birth. This should be a red flag that there is a problem in the core. Not plagiocephaly ... but a delay in the remolding of the head after birth ... at seventy-two hours the head should be remolded; for many, twenty-four hours is sufficient.

ONE BREATH

Practical

Evaluate the connection between the Movement of eternity, thoracic respiration, and Primary Respiration in an adult.

Is there One Breath?

TRANSMUTATION REVISITED

Transmutation is a very precise word. It means a complete change in the nature of something resulting in something of an entirely different nature. A change in the elemental. The change of one species into another. This word is misused so much that the reason Sutherland chose it may not make sense.

Transmutation is not transformation. It is much more profound. It is like changing silica into calcium or a criminal into a peaceful leader. Our goal here is to observe transmutation during treatment rather than its aftereffects. Let's review our prior discussions on transmutation in the courses.

In Phase One we discussed metabolic activity as the basis for cranial motion, rather than dural levers. The description of the metabolic process was as follows: The Breath of Life catalyzes motion by directing Its Potency into Its Creation. The Potency is a Fire that transmutes all substance as it acts. During the Inhalation Phase of Primary Respiration there is motion, which is an effect of the Potency of the Breath of Life. We can sense a variety of outcomes: Internal Disengagement, Internal Augmentation, Synchronization, Transmutation, and Reorientation to Midline. All these events are physiological and the result of the Tide's Potency transmuting inertial chemistry into motion and power that causes Life to move in the direction of ease, given to it by the space created of low tension. Space opens and function moves in ... this is Life.

This metabolic process comes from the Fire of Life, not a mechanical motion. The Fire burns away the old and recharges the whole. This transmutation can be seen directly. One can see the Fire and the lesion field and witness Tissue becoming Fluid, Fluid becoming soft potency, soft potency becoming Dynamic Stillness … et cetera … onward to the Health from whence it comes and to which it returns.

TRANSMUTATION

Practical

What happens when we move with the Transmutation, not behind it with the effects?

BALANCED RHYTHMIC INTERCHANGE

The term "balanced rhythmic interchange" was rarely used. The few who did use it were William Sutherland, Rollin Becker, and Robert Fulford ... I am sure there were others. No explanation was given ... for years I have loved the feeling of the words "balanced rhythmic interchange" as a precursor to the fusion of the yin and yang into the Sea of Wholeness. These are my thoughts from a biochemical point of view.

The ideal fluid body is something we can only imagine from the writings of our forefathers. But ... we can sense it in newborns and begin the journey from fragments to the whole. We have a sensation to remember ... a newborn fluid body, what a sacred fire ... so soft and luminous.

Then we see the distorted fluid body in ourselves. The journey from distortion to sacred function takes many years, as we ourselves limit the perception. As Rollin often said, "we must pull back the veil." Actually, the Tide heals us so we can see Love incarnating and pass into a non-dualistic world.

Wholeness is an ideal that has been glorified throughout the history of healing. Some teachers have come to realize this in themselves and have inspired others to seek what we call the Wholeness of the Health or the Oneness in which everything *is* the whole.

As Osteopaths, our journey begins with the diagnosis of disease/lesions. Lesions by their nature appear independent from the whole. When demoralization happens, we see only parts, i.e., pieces of reality with polarities. When aware of the whole, we cannot see pieces because the Ocean demonstrates an equalness to and in everything, a homogenous field.

Lesioning causes the parts to be unable to unite. This is a serious physiological loss that one must be aware of in Fluid Body Dynamics; that is to say, the chemistry cannot "work." This is called a Withering Field.

THE BUILDING OR REBUILDING OF PHYSIOLOGY

Wholeness is oneness. Oneness is part-less.

When lesioned, parts are separate and not united.

They are a duality … two independent distorted pieces.

There is no augmentation or meaningful communication.

Their fulcrums are separate.

When neutral occurs, everything is homogenized.

Then, during treatment, the original fulcrum of the function appears.

This is the future preceding the present into which the two become one.

As the treatment ensues, the two parts gather around the fulcrum of the

Oneness and are relieved of the distortions.

A lateral fluctuation occurs between the two separate parts around the center

point of the future chemistry.

This is balanced rhythmic interchange.

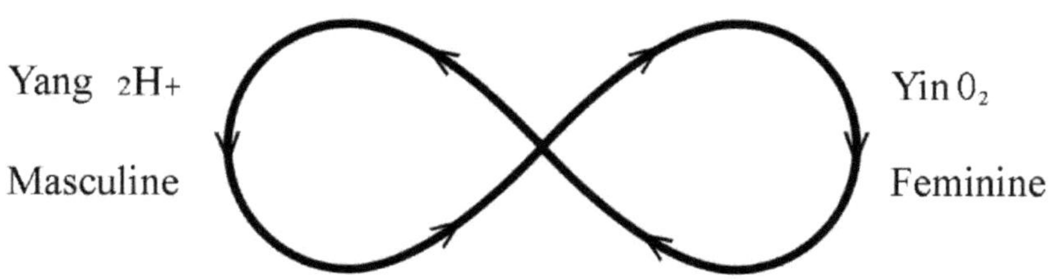

Then there is a stillness that suffuses the whole.

Then the neutral substance materializes as the original compound.

The two are gone … only the original compound exists.

The original compound is destined to serve not itself but the whole.

The opposite parts interface with the Tide through neutrality. Then the opposites balance around the common center (preexisting future / design of the Health). Then the process of balanced rhythmic interchange occurs as the lateral fluctuation around the center point and brings the transmutation of the opposites into union. The parts no longer exist with any of their prior being-ness—that is, their essence; now their identity has been transmuted into a new being-ness. So their essential nature has moved closer toward fruition. No memory of prior being-ness remains.

There is always a Third principle at work providing transmutation.

Tidal Transmutation is moving everything toward the upper circle. The healing process itself occurs around a fulcrum of the Wholeness that everything is moving toward, while creation moves from the upper circle into an incarnate form that can arise back to CAUSE.

HOMEOSTASIS

The Basis of Health

Homeostasis is a quintessential state of balance that allows adaptation of the whole organism to changing external and internal activities.

It is the innate neutral state of the whole.

This is a silent space where even synaptic noise is but a whisper. It is the basis of health in all healing arts ... the ability of the organism to adapt, act, and return to a balance point—that is, to automatically shift as it is moved by Life. Health could be described as the capacity to adapt to change ... it certainly is the definition of mental health.

How does normal become established ... where does this state of balance in the whole come from?

My understanding is this:

In the beginning, the supernatural Mind creates perfect Beingness as a whole. This is an Ocean radiating from its center. The center is silence and is everywhere in the Sea. This center is called the Health. It is the reference point for the whole of normal function.

The being-ness of all the essential parts forms as the whole unfolds.

The center point of all functions are joined in a wholeness that precedes the individual parts. The whole keeps the parts centered in a syncytium that mystifies the imagination. Sutherland said,

"When all the fulcrums are synchronized, there will be peace and harmony."

Appreciation of the Fluid Body as one drop cascades us into a "relative whole" through which the parts can augment each other within a synchronized Whole. This elevated view of the organism is Osteopathic thinking that reflects the interface of many true sciences.

"You are a drop that contains an Ocean, not a drop in the Ocean." –Rumi

Normal persists because of homeostasis. Homeostasis is maintained through the activity of automatic shifting, an intrinsic capacity to transmute any tensions, which inhibit the return to balance around the preestablished center point of the Whole.

We studied this in the early Phases. We witnessed automatic shifting and stillpoints that radiated into the Sea Around Us. Unfortunately for humans, the return to our "Sea of Origin" requires a neutral emotional and mental state from which the automatic shifting of perception can occur and lift the veil that keeps our awareness in smaller circles and at faster tempos.

By balancing the whole, we enable the parts to return to homeostasis (neutral).

When we understand all this, we see how Sutherland's work with Primary Respiration can bring incredible results ... This kind of thinking is very scientific and yet is difficult for many physicians to believe: if they address the whole, the part will heal ... this is so scientific that I am amazed at how we can avoid the Truth ...

Each function or structure has a point of balance within itself. For example, every tissue form (anatomy) starts from a point, an embryonic seed (primordium). This point is the doorway to unfoldment, renewal, and healing. It is the center point for spatial activity (range of motion). It is also the center point for the physiological network. Every form or function has a balance point for rest and homoeostasis. It must return to its origin to drink from the waters of Life that replenish its entirety, even its Self.

Any function can express a physical or physiological range of normal metabolic motion. For example, calcium activity has a balance point that determines in some perfect manner the fulcrum for the range of function. This normal range of activity is chemical. Intrinsically, then, we have a range of normal around a center point, which forms the shape of the function and its range of normal metabolic movement that makes mechanical movement possible. Outside the "norm," the parts dysfunction.

Biomechanical laws are expressions of physiology, not isolated mechanical actions like we see in a machine. This has been all but forgotten. For example, place your elbow on a table and rest your chin on your hand ... feel the biceps muscle ... it should feel ... like a bag of "fluid" standing and waiting but not dead. Waiting is a state of being available to respond ... this neutrality allows the function to hear and receive the command. Then there is action, which is a physiological process.

Our physiology needs neutrality; it is a time when there is exchange within all the fluids of the body ... when homeostasis occurs.

Still's use of the term "withering field" for a lesion is ingenious, as it reflects the above principles at the most essential level of being. The quality of a function is in proportion to its capacity for neutrality. This also occurs in perceptual activity.

Mental neutrality is a mind at rest, a mind at peace and alert to instruction from the Supreme Intelligence that creates and sustains us. A neutral mind can listen without cataloguing the data given to it. The response is immediate and full but lacks the rigidity of a plan. It is the direction of ease.

Without neutrality, we become compromised and apathetic

toward others, whom we judge through projections from the rational mind. The world is a war of opposites, not "equalnesses."

We see neutral all the time ... we call it Beauty.

The temple bell stops

But the sound keeps coming

Out of the flowers

–Matsuo Basho (17th Century)

As we begin our perceptual journey in this phase of our life, we begin listening with all of our senses.

This is a hard transition.

AUTONOMIC BALANCE

Homeostasis or neutral in a function reflects autonomic balance in that function.

When we feel autonomic imbalance in an organ, neutral can be restored to change the function considerably.

For example, one senses sympathetic tension in kidney function. This tension is functional, not organic; it can cause malaise. Unresolved, it can lead to disease. If the neutral balance can be restored, its chemical milieu will change for the better.

FROM OSTEOPATHY

The term "neutral," or "idling," has been in our vocabulary since Fryette's Laws were proposed circa 1916. His observation of neutral was that the state of normal for any structure/function is neutrality, with neutral being a state of "standing stoppage," so to speak, because the function is waiting to act, that is, idling like an engine, waiting for the command to move into action obediently in response to the mind of the whole: "the engine of Life" ... as Still liked to call it.

HOMEOSTASIS

Homeostatsis is when a dynamically stable state is maintained in a system. There may be disturbances from external forces, in which case internal processes regulate and counteract them.

In the physiology of the body, relatively constant conditions are maintained as a result of homeostasis.

The word is derived from "homeo" which means "like" and "stasis" which means "stoppage".

Homeostasis literally means a standing stoppage in a physiological process, but the stop is powerful vitality, not lassitude.

THE MEETING PLACE AND EROS

The Meeting Place is a special landscape for us. It blossoms into something unexpected and universal.

The meeting place is not an end in itself.

One can easily go there and not change. The observer can easily "look for something to happen"; this has the effect of a mirror ... and nothing will grow. In all our work we must be careful to listen deeply without looking. This silent activity can be delayed by one trying to experience something. One must keep alert for what one cannot conceive of and listen with devotion ... to have the mind of a child whose heart is innocent and sacred.

The emptiness that births the True Self is an effect of realizing our ignorance/dependence. Out of respect for the Tide and God, we do not assume the capacity to know or see. Knowing and seeing do happen in the natural world to a limited extent, but the meeting place is the edge of the supernatural world. Here the meeting only comes when we listen; listen into the silence with full faith ... the "other" will come.

Third level stillness is not an end in itself ... not something to hold onto but something to be in and become from.

Both the Meeting Place and Third Level Stillness are birthing rooms where one's individuality merges into a new form of being. To be specific, one experiences Eros. Eros is the unity that promotes the meeting and merger necessary for further growth. Eros is originally from the Greek, Plato in particular. Later, Carl Jung, Rollo May, and Helen Luke referred often to Eros as a specific state of being. Modern-day language associates Eros with a sexual event. This is far from the truth and very tragic, as potentialities are stripped away by contemporizing the word for the ego.

When you come to see how this word connects one with the true nature of love, you may feel awed.

This Platonic love (Eros) is rare because one is giving endlessly rather than having a need met and coming to an end or climax. This love springs from awe of the "other." One merges. The sense of "me" or "I" is literally mixed with the other and a true sense of new being is established. It is born into wholeness so simple that diversity ends and for a period there is nothing but the unity of all ... this replaces the "others" with a singular identity homogenized into a single ONE. The transparency of the ONENESS is a silent love that leads by its own will to an end of "I" as one has known it in many forms of individual will ... One's individuality dies as one comes to rest in the Beloved Mystery of Life.

Eros can occur, as we said, between souls. It can also be a merger with a body of true knowledge ... This is not an everyday thought for educated people.

Knowledge that precedes mankind's appearance in time is supernatural.

The principles in Osteopathy predate A. T. Still. The Breath of Life, the Tide, Silence, and Stillness are all preincarnate laws, as are embryology, transmutation, and Health. Love of these realities can lead to awe and merger. The individual becomes the knowledge that he or she partners with.

One gives one's being to the Wisdom without a need for return, because the giving first comes from a truth which echoes in the heart eternally. This can lead to the same consummation as in the other forms of Eros ... arrival at the doorway to heaven or God's presence ... then a new Self, a True Self, journeys as a Wholeness into the Sun.

The ego is a self-centered event and cannot meet the "other" without taking for its own need. We can hold at a third level stillness and believe it is "higher" ... The ego must love enough to die. The coming of Eros into one's arena is a surprise ... one is bewildered at the giving without conditional needs. The expression is spontaneous ... it goes on forever in a landscape of awe and surprise.

This change makes one unpredictable to others, but to the new Self the unpredictable is the constant motion of Life and its spontaneous Tide.

Love of this kind is ever full and ever new.

Trust in the Tide has become one's livingness. The ease is filled with the unexpected expansion of the wholeness as previously experienced. Often the Love itself coming from God loses its individual intonations ... only the whole can be loved ... not me ... everything and everyone as a whole.

Knowing where you are is easy ... what's missing is "Me" and duality ... any movement into diversity is isolating and cold.

The language used in the Biodynamic view of Osteopathy is classical, not contemporary. Sutherland was a wordsmith; his language was very specific. Words are created and incarnate through specific observers. The words tell us what they observed. Serene is a huge word, huge. Transmutation, likewise, is supernatural. If you try to see the word in action, you will perhaps return to Cause.

The First Clue that Eros is coming is when we see God in the face of another ... a light suffusing us.

Remember ... Dr. Still said, "I love my patients because I see God in their faces and form." This is not imagination.

Some of the qualities of Eros are listed below:

It is a becoming of being in a new Self through merger

It binds diversity into wholeness

It is the yearning for wholeness, continually

It leaps barriers between enemies

It drives one to transcend oneself

It is the source of tenderness

It requires divergent imagination

It transcends technique in any form

It loves humanity

It receives as the whole of life receives

It follows

The Meeting Place is where one listens. As this occurs, therein is maturation. The heart becomes neutral and is receptive to the Tide, which creates merger.

During maturation, one rests in a loving presence.

Here the senses convert to seeing the whole rather than the singular.

Soon one comes to see the Given as all there is.

Little if any effort is made to actualize ... to be.

The Known becomes a secret.

An inner voice appears as the Teacher.

One follows the Mystery.

THE POTENCY OF THE TIDE IS FIRE

"Fire is in all things

Pervades all things without intermingling with them

Shining by its very nature, hidden

Manifesting its presence only when it can find material to work on

Violent and invisible

Having absolute rule over all things

It comprehends but remains incomprehensible

Never in need

Mysteriously increasing itself

Showing forth the nature of its Majesty, according to the nature of the substance receiving it

Powerful and Mighty

Invisibly present in all things."

–Dionysius (first century AD, Christian mystic, first Bishop of Athens, friend of Paul and the Disciples, met with Mary, was a spiritual father to many)

THE MOVEMENT OF FIRE

This practical will review many of the basic motions related to Primary Respiration that we have all learned from a variety of courses in traditional cranial work.

Fire is essential to being. Fire is the nature of the Potency and the potency with different levels of transmutative intensity. Transmutation is more than the effect of fire as we generally appreciate it in science. The Tidal Fire destroys and rebuilds. It is the force that generates growth and development. It carries the Mind of God into manifestation. It expresses the Health and its Liquid Light. It burns away the dross of the ego.

It is the Breathing of the rates. Fire brings shape and boundary into the function it creates. Breathing Fire, Transmutation, Metabolic Motion, Form, Death, Rebuilding, Healing, and Heat are all little pieces of the flame visible at different moments. It can stop at Will. It's not wildfire. It can pause, melt into neutral, or go still, holding its power in the whole as a new beingness. It comes from the Spark that ignites the engine of life. It is Holy Fire. It is Love.

FIRE

Practical

We will look again at all we know and see what is now visible that was before invisible.

Begin with a bowl of water, as we did in Phase One …

a transparent bowl of fluid …

The Fire comes and there is a change.

THE FLAME OF INTENTION

One of Dr. Sutherland's goals was to communicate with the Tide. As you know, he labored long and hard to free himself from the "physical senses," as he called them. As he did, new horizons opened. He began to recognize the Tide as an effect of a Supreme and Loving Intelligence. He then understood that the Will and Intention of God could be realized.

This awakening did not occur overnight; it was the effect of a great effort to think independently of what he knew. It was also the outcome of faith in the Tide and being neutral enough to let it enter him.

Thinking Osteopathy leads us into new landscapes. As we enter these places, we are healed by the Presence of the Tide. This healing changes our senses from a materialistic reductionist convergent function into senses reconnected to the Health, and we see life in a very different way. As this change occurs, we begin at times to see that the world is transparent to the Breath of Life ... that everything is moving from one eternal source, Love and Creation eternally in motion. This realization is a Beautiful shock, one that changes our Thinking and our sense of normality.

These changes are not automatic; one must wish for less internal chaos and want to be healed. This requires a practical faith in the Tide, which is a trust that allows change, change that is not predictable. The ego in its laziness will resist, and so it takes many years to find oneself empty of willfulness and filled with a soft joy, silence, peace, and neutrality.

A relationship with the Mover of the Tide helps many patients who would otherwise benefit much less from any method available in medicine today. It also allows entry into the world of children that is clinically miles ahead of the more rigid formats.

Now we will work with the "Flame of Intention." It is a therapeutic force that can be seen in every patient (as the Tide permits). It can communicate to us the Intention of the Breath of Life. It also reveals a precise look at its laser-like "noninvasive surgical skill" at a cellular level. The flame will communicate its Intention clearly and will demonstrate that Intention without you adding any intention of your own other than attentiveness to the Flame.

The intention is not a conclusion from what you see but a transmission from the Wisdom of the Flame.

THE FLAME

Practical

Notice that everything is Transparent to the Breath of Life. There is a wind passing through everything. It is the motion of Creation, the eternal motion of Divine Love.

If this is not easily noticed, look outside in Nature for a while, then at the patient, with divergent vision—vision that does not focus anywhere. If this does not help, sit in Third Level Stillness for a while and let it help you to a neutrality of the senses.

Trust your judgment. If it is a fantasy, then the treatment will not work. Take the risk to trust what you see and embrace it.

Go to the patient and place your hands on the flame. Make sensory contact and mold your hands to the shape, with the longest fingers abutting the tip of the flame.

Physically follow the Flame and listen to it ... focus your attention with great care.

It will demonstrate a treatment at many levels.

It will stop without making the patient perfect.

The flame does not go out but recedes into a liquid light.

Let the patient rest.

THE CENTRAL NERVOUS SYSTEM DIAGNOSTICS

Each separate activity is evaluated for the following:

Internal disengagement under the influence of the Tide

Synchronization with the Tide (check for paradoxical motion)

Augmentation with other motions of the system (check for contradictory motions)

Transmutation of the function toward neutral

Activities to evaluate:

The sacs (periosteal, dural, brain proper)

The neural tube

Bowing of the tadpole into the Sea around Us

The Tadpole as a whole moving toward lamina terminalis during inhalation (only with rates)

Coiling in the lateral ventricles toward lamina terminalis during the inhalation period

Rocking on the waterbeds

The Bird

Ignition: Motion Present of reciprocal tension potency in the third ventricle

Central nervous system Fluid Field

Central nervous system collective reciprocal tension potency

WHAT'S AT THE BOTTOM OF A SEAM

When we truly enter a seam, there is only Space. There is no sense of a space in between layers of anatomy. In the seam we enter a Dynamic Stillness. It is like a deep dark well.

One cannot tell where the bottom is ... we move deeper into the well.

It is dark.

Eventually, we come to the bottom.

Find a comfortable spot and Rest ... wait for the dawn.

When the dawn comes, you will see the landscape at the bottom of the Seam ...

Rebalance if necessary ... Zone B, the Ocean, and the doorway between them ... or go to the Health and wait (preferred method).

Further Comments on Seams

The essential feature of a seam is space, but not the space between anatomical landmarks. Space is a specific state of Life in which functions the invisible matrix of the Health.

Space is bigger than the function it creates.

Therapeutic forces recognize seams as they frequently disappear into a seam before the seams merge into pure space.

The therapeutic forces one engages in a seam vary from the Long-Tide and the Dynamic Stillness to the Liquid Light of the Health.

Space is a rich dark substance. Still said, "Life is that substance which fills all the spaces of the universe."

IF

If you sense a Living patient under your hands, and if you sense the Health first, and if you synchronize with Beauty before the Lesion, and if you are a true scientist without bias, and if you listen instead of Speak with your hands, and if you can wait for your mind to be Neutral, and if you are not distracted by former skill, and if you are not trying to fix only the Symptoms, and if you can see the direction of ease, and if you understand Dr. Still's first chapter in *Philosophy of Osteopathy*, and if you believe that your hands can show you more than you can show them, and if you believe that your job is to follow and not to lead the Mechanism of Life, and if you can look for something new in each treatment, and if you are trying to cooperate with Laws not framed by human hands, and if you believe that Life is Eternal, and if you burn all the books once you have a foundation, and if you can enter the wilderness inside yourself and the patient, and if you believe Love is the Cause of everything, and if you can take opposition without resistance, and if your mind wants to be Transparent to your own Health, and if your Ignorance does not hide but becomes humble, and if you see all forms of Osteopathy as branches on one tree, and if you have read Sutherland again and again and again, and if you see that Thoracic Respiration Neutrals are a priori to a Complete Neutral, and if you know that there is no form without formlessness and no Life without Death, Transmutation, and Renewal, and if you know that the treatment is already waiting in the patient, and if you know that your help is what is needed for a hundred reasons, and if you know we only help the treatment begin, and if you know that it is self-sustaining, and if you can love people who destroy the treatment before they leave the office, and if you do not expect more from yourself than what God grants you, and if you know you must leave everything you know behind in the dust of yesterday, and if you know stillness is not Stillness, and if you teach only from what you love, and if you can be fearlessly Neutral in your heart and breathe, and if you can feel the Health when you cannot feel it … Then, my friend, you will be a Joyful Beginner Osteopath. Then, if you wish, your prayers will be answered.

CLINICIAN'S STATE OF MIND

Thoracic Respiration as Cranial Rhythmic Impulse	2.5 cycles per minute (24 sec. per cycle)	6 cycles per ten minutes (100 sec. per cycle	Dynamic Stillness no perceivable rate·	Ocean of Love
Distracted with concepts	Urban mind ... insecurity; Attention; efferent; Forceful goals	The Mind settled by the Long-Tide; Natural mind Afferent	The mind Is waiting for the Tide; Neutral disciplined mind	True Self .... Light leads awareness
Mind full of thoughts, noisy, lesion oriented	Mind quiets but one Is vulnerable to fear	Mind is stable, pliable, and attentive; trust awakens	Wholeness is appreciated	Service of Inner child
Rational format – find lesion and resolve it	Self serving goals; Co-dependency; subjective analysis	Instinctive awareness of a Greater Mind	The Mystery is evident; Senses rest and convert	One Is fulfilled; Health rises to surface ...
Emotionally unstable, Self -Centered	Empathy Is a challenge; Fluctuations appear	Response to the Tide begins ...	Rest; maturation	Alignment with the will of the Tide
Little sense of inner dynamics in self or patient; lesion Is antagonist	Sensitivity present but undisciplined; Moments of Insecurity and trust vacillate	Instinct awakens; attention softens; feminine appears	Conversion of the senses to invisible world	Nothingness
Breathing is not synchronized with other rhythms; Sympathetic Breathing	Breathing begins to change	Synchronization or breathing with the Tide	Breaths unite	Cause of Breath Is Love
Observer is fixed on Goal; Intentions are fixed	Observer Is left-brained	Observer is neutral	Observer moved by Tide	The Original Observer
Attention focal	Attention shifts with fluid	Attention Is open	Sense of Self is the whole	Attention Is given

"Let That From Which You Were Wounded Become Your Cure." –Migne

"A mechanic in the science of knowing is able to perceive the Tide in operation ... if Knowing and the Tide are synonymous, then, as these patients come to me for observation, diagnosis, and treatment, and I am aware of an underlying quality of activity taking place beyond the fulcrums and patterns, at times during their stay in the office, momentary periods of Stillness occur depending on the problem, and in a few minutes the material picture changes considerably, and always toward freedom. The important point I am trying to state is that this underlying Tide is universal, without definition, and has no real connection to the problems. Like the glasshouse described in Kirksville. 'The Breath of Life or Tide does not touch the house but lights it up by reflecting through and through.'" –R. Becker, *The Stillness of Life*, p. 208.

"Life is that calm force sent forth by Deity to vivify all of nature." –A. T. Still

"When embryonic respiration is restored, it neither gathers nor scatters, is without self or other [duality] ... it unites the yin and the yang." –Zhao Bi-Chen (19th-century Daoist Master)

MAMMALIAN EMBRYOGENESIS

As a principle of physics, all movements occur in relation to a reference point. This is especially important in an expanding mass such as an embryo, since all structures not attached to the surface understandably move away from the surface as the mass expands. Under such conditions, the ideal reference point would be one in the center of the mass, i.e., a centroid. Even though no such consistently occurring point exists in developing embryos, any point that is more centrally located would move less in relation to surrounding structures ...

The definitive locations of the internal structures ... can be explained by differential growth. ... Rather than structures moving from one region of the embryo to another, ... they spread out within the same region, as the embryo enlarges and changes shape.

Raymond F. Gasser PhD,
full article:
https://anatomypubs.onlinelibrary.wiley.com/doi/full/10.1002/ar.b.20092

A Biodynamic view of Osteopathy in the cranial field appreciates the movement of wholeness around, through, and within the fulcrum of the wholeness of Primary Respiration. This understanding is reflected in the word Biodynamic, which, in the context of this original Osteopathic model, means that the organism is emerging from its most intimate and central creative fulcrum, which is the Wholeness of the sea around us, through us, and in us of which we are an expression.

Therefore, in our teaching we approach this movement of the whole of the patient in the same way as Dr. Gasser presents it in his image of his "sense" of creation.

It is interesting that Dr. Gasser's recent work validates the exact point that has been of central interest to many Osteopaths for many, many years. And so, we again see that our research, by means of simple and skillful observation, is as accurate as, and perhaps more evolved than, the use of instrumentation. My point is that we need to trust what we feel and share it with others, and over a period of time new principles of treatment will continue to unveil themselves from the Truth that is already there.

THE PARABLE OF THE TARES, FROM MATTHEW 13:24–30, KJV

24 Another parable put he forth unto them, saying, The
kingdom of heaven is likened unto a man which sowed good
seed in his field:
25 But while men slept, his enemy came and sowed tares
among the wheat, and went his way.
26 But when the blade was sprung up, and brought forth
fruit, then appeared the tares also.
27 So the servants of the householder came and said unto
him, Sir, didst not thou sow good seed in thy field? from
whence then hath it tares?
28 He said unto them, An enemy hath done this. The
servants said unto him, Wilt thou then that we go and gather
them up?
29 But he said, Nay; lest while ye gather up the tares, ye root
up also the wheat with them.
30 Let both grow together until the harvest: and in the time
of harvest I will say to the reapers, Gather ye together first the
tares, and bind them in bundles to burn them: but gather the
wheat into my barn.

Commentary

The Kingdom of Heaven is the place of good wheat and the finest bread, The Bread of Life.

It's the holy ground of union with God, of Love Eternal. A place of being far beyond our imagination and comprehension. Beyond Miracles, the place where Miracles come from.

The good seed is our Imago Dei, the Health. "Good seed" in the agricultural area of the time would be perfectly clean, not mixed with the seeds of weeds. It also means that the seed was fresh and from healthy plants that were immune to local diseases. It could withstand the weeds that the enemy threw next to the good seed, and still ripen alongside them, without loss.

The workers wanted to get rid of the weeds right away, to pull them up and get rid of them. The Master said, Wait. Let them grow. Wait until the Wheat matures. If you pull out the weeds now, you will damage the growth and development of the wheat.

The sense here is that we can be patient, wait, and if the seed is healthy, it will not be diminished by the weeds.

Later, when the wheat is full, the weeds can be pulled, burned (transmuted), and the wheat stored as Memory Eternal, the true wheat (source of nourishment) from the seed of Love.

What Christ may be pointing to is nonviolence, Neutrality toward the enemy and the weeds ... applied to meditation, it could mean that we do not remove lesions but continue to grow with weeds ... If we pull out lesions before the harvest is met, then the Wholeness suffers. The good is damaged ... so at Harvest, when we are with the Health, and mature, the weeds will be pulled and transmuted.

The crop (being in the Heart of the Health) can be stored (memory eternal) for our nourishment.

It is amazing how often Teachers move us away from self-improvement by the use of forceful rejection of the undesirable aspects of our Humanity ... and how often the desire to pull them out comes along. Christ suggests another road.

Illness is often seen as a weed. If one waits and lets the Health grow, the time will come when the Fire will consume the weeds in

Compassion … not to reject the weeds but to change them into something that supports the Health.

Overzealous correction of lesions can damage Wholeness.

DOCTOR STILL'S PRAYER

Lord, great healer, I kneel before You.
Since excellent grace and perfect gifts descend from You, grant, I implore You, ability to my hands, lucidity to my intelligence,
kindness and empathy in my heart.
Give me simplicity of purpose, the strength to bring to my hands part of the burden of my suffering brothers, and a real understanding of the privilege You have given me.
Remove from my heart all malice and prejudice,

so that with sincere childish faith I
can lean on You, Amen.

Andrew Taylor Still

Autobiography of Andrew T. Still (Revised Edition, 1908).

THE SIMPLICITY OF OSTEOPATHY

Osteopathy is as simple as the human organism, and that is as simple as the universe, for in the human organism are embraced all the physical, mental and spiritual laws of the universe.

To perfectly understand the human organism then, it would be necessary to possess an infinite mind.

...we are prone to forget that the body must cure itself. That is the osteopathic idea, and in that there is a simplicity.

We should aid the body in every spiritual, mental, biological and physiological way possible, but there is no doubt in my mind that the structural aspect is of prime importance....

...if we compare our diagnosis and therapy to that of the M.D.'s, our methods are much more simple in a large majority of cases, for there is a mechanical factor in almost every case that is over-looked by them, and we may be sure if these mechanical factors are removed, the patient will do better than he did before....

The principle of osteopathy is simple, as all great truths are simple. Its application is not. It requires infinite pains.

Harrison H. Fryette, "The Simplicity of Osteopathy," in *American Academy of Osteopathy,* 1938, p. 14–15.

"To carry the self forward and illuminate myriad things is delusion.

That myriad things come forth and illuminate the self is awakening."

Dōgen Zenji

This is from the essay titled Genjōkōan (often translated as "Actualizing the Fundamental Point").

It was originally written in 1233.

BIODYNAMICS OF OSTEOPATHY BOOK SERIES

This book is one of a series of twelve *Biodynamics of Osteopathy* books. It is recommended that you read the whole series in order, as each book builds on the understanding from prior books. It is also recommended that you seek experienced teachers and mentors to help you experience the full depth of the information given.

The full series is as follows:

Phase One is about involuntary motion, which is motion present in the whole and in the lesion. We learn to synchronize with the breathing of Primary Respiration before we approach any treatment. This synchronization is the key to working with stable rates and not irritating the system. The principle of synchronizing with a healthy aspect of the patient suffuses the whole teaching program. This synchronization shifts our awareness to a different level of receptivity, which allows us to see Primary Respiration rather than the lesion field, and this eventually leads us to an understanding of the intention of Primary Respiration.

Phase Two is about communication with the natural laws of healing that surround activity at 2 to 3 cycles per minute. We synchronize with the breathing of Primary Respiration and also add the skill of sensing the fulcrum, the Stillness through which the breathing creates form and function. It is a different kind of synchronization from that in Phase One, shifting our awareness more deeply. As this occurs, the treatment automatically expresses itself. The end point of treatment, when compared with Phase One, reveals several differences. We find this kind of synchronization works exclusively with the fluid body and the outcome of treatment is more complete than when working with tissue alone.

Phase Three is centered around the activities of the Long Tide (100 second cycle). We explore an indwelling therapeutic force already present in the lesion field. We learn that the dural system is not made-up of three sickles but rather a series of folds in a sac, arising during growth and development. We see the relationship between the upper and lower dural sacs, awakening us to the independence of two separate tentorium cerebelli. We discover that zone D, the horizon, and the Wire (along which the Long Tide moves during its intended therapeutic course) are all linked as natural laws pertaining to this level of Primary Respiration.

Phase Four focuses on the Midline, a place where the spatial relationships are expressed as a whole. It synchronizes and centers us in such a way that we become aware of Zone D and the Dynamic Stillness. The Third Level Stillness in Phase Four is different from the Stillness in the other Phases – we are centered by the Stillness at the center of creation. Our intention is replaced by the intention of the Tide which can facilitate our spiritual path.

Phase Five is about *the face*. As we approach the face, we use all of the principles that we have learned in Phase One, Two, Three, and Four. We work with automatic shifting and notice differences from how the face is viewed by older models within Osteopathy in the Cranial Field. As we synchronize with the therapeutic presence of the Long Tide we see what we can learn about the face from that landscape. We also work with Seams, Dynamic Stillness, and Ignition.

Phase Six is a continuation of our journey into the Wholeness that generates life and delivers therapeutic forces that transmute lesions once Neutral is expressed. It is a mixture of activities centered around the outside presence of Primary Respiration as something that is a non-biological force and that has a persona. We will also continue to explore seams and then move on to the extremities, first in the embryological terms and then as Sutherland taught them in his work called PowerPoints. Phase 6 is a time to build your understanding of the Tide and refine your skills.

Phase Seven highlights the Health. Dr. Still's famous comment "Find the Health; anyone can find disease," has plagued many minds over the last century. We come to the clear vision of several indwelling aspects of the Health: Love ... liquid light ... and a diamond matrix. A approach to the terminally ill and dying patient is addressed. In the somatic sensation of the Tide passing through the House Under the Sea, our awareness is transmuted by the Health. The lesion is seen as a precognitive act of the Health. Thoracic Respiration, Primary Respiration, and Ignition are as One. The landscape is vast ... and the principles of healing are even more substantial than we have previously experienced..

Phase Eight is a deeper exploration of seams, balanced rhythmic interchange, and the Flame of Intention as a therapeutic modality. Phase Eight is the culmination of our awareness of Wholeness, and ultimately brings us to the Divine Presence, Unconditional Love and Oneness. The living Tide dominates the awareness while forms move to the background. One feels the Breath of Creation in oneself as the Center of Wholeness. One feels the Unfoldment of oneself as one is Created. Our consciousness is a gift; we do not own it and if we try to control it we lose Wholeness.

Phase Nine is when we are able to fully evaluate and treat the Central Nervous System and the Eye. We also address Fire and the therapeutic modality of the Shakedown. True action is moved from Love and makes our perception exist. This Love is self-emptying and by its nature allows us to Serve as part of the Perfect. Perception can be used to Serve something other than ourselves. We have attempted to enter this balance point between the Perfect and the Disease ... it is a point where the whole of everything is suspended by Love as it works to incarnate the Complete. In the balance point of everything is The Intention of the Tide following the movement of the distortion back to a True relationship with the Blueprint of Life.

Pediatrics One explores how children grow as a whole, not in parts as we sometimes believe. Children live in the Direction of Ease of motion present in their fluid metabolic fields, otherwise they get uncomfortable and require assistance. Does your treatment directly support the whole, or does it assume to support the whole? We realize children are not adults and cannot be treated as adults are. We approach the therapeutic modality of the "Meeting Place", prenatal and postnatal periods, the treatment of the pelvis during pregnancy, fetal malposition and labor.

Pediatrics Two is where we deepen in the perceptive awareness necessary to approach the treatment of children. We deepen in our appreciation of Wholeness, the three levels of Stillness and the "Meeting Place". We approach "Desert Neutral", where therapeutics pass into the neutral substance, and a mystery unfolds as the breath of Divine love cascades as a therapeutic force across a night desert landscape, filling and leaving behind no visible effects. We further address treatment of the pelvis and the uterus during pregnancy. We explore thoracic and Primary Respiration in children, and the Family Circle.

Pediatrics Three is where we continue to study the therapeutic Flow of Attention. We deepen in Third Level Stillness and the Meeting Place. The Meeting Place is easily misinterpreted ... our observer must be so still and neutral that the process can be seen as it happens. The central nervous system in the child can be finally approached for evaluation and treatment. We explore teething and also the "locked up head". We use the therapeutic modality of the Flame of Intention, and its connection to the Breath of Life. Everything is transparent to the Breath of Life.

ABOUT THE AUTHOR

James Jealous, D.O. (1943–2021), was an osteopathic physician, teacher, and writer. His life's work was founding and developing **Biodynamics of Osteopathy**, a unique methodology he established within the field of osteopathy, following the lineage of Dr. A.T. Still and Dr. W.G. Sutherland.

He was born in Saco, Maine, and since his father was an osteopathic physician, he was around osteopathy from an early age. He studied at Kirksville College of Osteopathic Medicine in Missouri (now the A.T. Still University of Health Sciences), graduating in 1970. He then set up practice in rural Maine as an osteopathic primary care physician.

Over time, Dr. Jealous saw parallels between the work of embryologist Dr. Erich Blechschmidt and that of osteopathic physician Dr. William Garner Sutherland. This inspiration led him to create his own body of work. In the early 1990s, he began teaching "A Biodynamic View of Osteopathy in the Cranial Field," which, as he developed his specific methodology, was refined to "Biodynamics of Osteopathy."

A deeply spiritual person, he felt most at home in the natural world and was an avid fisherman and hiker.

For more information, please visit:
https://BiodynamicsOfOsteopathy.com

There is a wind passing through ...
it is the motion of creation,
the eternal motion of Divine love.